A COMPREHENSIVE GLUTEN & DAIRY FREE GROCERY LIST

Over 1000 Food Items From Every Department

Paula C. Henderson

A COMPREHENSIVE GLUTEN & DAIRY FREE GROCERY LIST

Book Title Copyright © 2019 by Paula C. Henderson. All Rights Reserved.

All rights reserved. No part of this book may be reproduced in any form or by any electronic or mechanical means including information storage and retrieval systems, without permission in writing from the author. The only exception is by a reviewer, who may quote short excerpts in a review.

Cover designed by Paula C. Henderson

Paula C. Henderson
Visit my website at www.Glutenfree-Dairyfree-Recipes.com

Printed in the United States of America

First Printing: July 2019

Paperback ISBN- 9781098618087

A COMPREHENSIVE GLUTEN & DAIRY FREE GROCERY LIST

CONTENTS

Contents

A COMPREHENSIVE GLUTEN & DAIRY FREE GROCERY LIST 1
CONTENTS 3
about this list 7
BAKING AISLE 8
BEVERAGES 11
BREAD 14
BOXED MIXES, ICING & PIE 16
BREAKFAST 18
    CEREAL 19
CANNED FOODS 20
    Canned and Dried Beans 20
    Canned and Packaged Meats/Seafoods 21
    Canned and Packaged Vegetables 23
    Canned and Packaged Fruits 24
    Canned Other 24
CONDIMENTS 25
    BARBECUE SAUCE 25
    Dressing 25
    MISCELLANEOUS 27
    SALSA 28
    SOY SAUCE & OTHER ASIAN SAUCES 29
    VINEGAR 29
FRUIT: produce 30
FROZEN FOODS 32
    BREAKFAST 32

A COMPREHENSIVE GLUTEN & DAIRY FREE GROCERY LIST

    DESSERTS 33
    ENTREES 34
    FRUITS 36
    MISCELLANEOUS 36
    PIZZA 36
    POTATOES 37
    VEGETABLES 37
MEAT AND SEAFOOD DEPARTMENT 38
MISCELLANEOUS 41
NUTS AND SEEDS 42
PACKAGED FOODS 43
PASTA, GRAINS, RICE, BOXED POTATOES 44
REFRIGERATED 45
    DAIRY FREE BUTTER SUBSTITUTES 46
    LUNCHMEAT 46
SHELF STABLE ENTREES 47
SNACK FOODS 48
    COOKIES AND SNACK CAKES 51
SOUPS, BROTHS, SAUCE AND GRAVY 52
    BROTH 52
    SOUP, CHILI, AND STEW 53
    GRAVY 53
    SAUCE 54
Spices & seasonings 55
SWEETENERS 58
VEGETABLES: produce 59
TIPS FOR HEALTHY GROCERY SHOPPING 61
RESOURCES FOR MORE INFORMATION 63

A COMPREHENSIVE GLUTEN & DAIRY FREE GROCERY LIST

SOME PRODUCT ARE GLUTEN FREE BUT NOT DAIRY FREE, AND VICE-VERSA. ONLY PRODUCTS THAT ARE BOTH GLUTEN AND DAIRY FREE BOTH ARE INCLUDED IN THIS LIST

A COMPREHENSIVE GLUTEN & DAIRY FREE GROCERY LIST

A COMPREHENSIVE GLUTEN & DAIRY FREE GROCERY LIST

ABOUT THIS LIST

This list of food products are a result of my literally reading the label of each item. However, you should always be suspect of any product that is packaged with an ingredient list as each brand may vary. Brands often change their ingredient lists – IMPROVED! NEW! So always check the label.

Many people can eat foods without direct gluten or dairy ingredients in the product. Others are so sensitive that they can have a reaction to foods that are naturally gluten and dairy free but were processed in a plant that also processes gluten and dairy food products. This is due to cross contamination.

If you are sensitive to cross contamination you should immediately stop eating any food if you have a bad reaction to the food. The most common foods exposed to cross contamination are grains like rice, corn, cornmeal, and oats. These foods are naturally gluten free but some do experience cross contamination from wheat flours processed in the same plant.

This is by no means ALL the foods! But, I hope this is a broad enough list to help you shop a little easier.

The following ingredients are gluten-free: Caramel color, Dextrin (controversial!!), Distilled Vinegar (not malt vinegar), maltose, maltodextrin, natural flavors and yeast extract. Even if you have not been diagnosed with Celiac, the Celiac.org website is a great reference for all things gluten free. If any of these ingredients cause you problems please omit it from your diet.

Be suspicious of the ingredient chocolate rather than cocoa. Cocoa is dairy free but not all chocolate is dairy free.

Other ingredients often found in gluten and dairy free products you may be sensitive to would be potato starch and soy ingredients.

SOME PRODUCT ARE GLUTEN FREE BUT NOT DAIRY FREE, AND VICE-VERSA. ONLY PRODUCTS THAT ARE BOTH GLUTEN AND DAIRY FREE ARE INCLUDED IN THIS LIST.

BAKING AISLE

> *Some gluten free boxed mixes, like some cake mixes, although gluten free, will have dairy so be sure to check the ingredient list. This list is both gluten and dairy free.*

1. 4c Gluten Free Plain Bread Crumbs
2. Albers Yellow Corn Meal
3. All-Purpose Gluten Free Flour
4. Almond Flour
5. Almond Milk, Shelf Stable
6. Almond Oil
7. Amaranth Flour
8. Arrowhead Mills Organic Gluten Free Brown Rice Flour
9. Arrowroot
10. Avocado Oil
11. Bakers Premium Unsweetened Chocolate Baking Bar
12. Baking Powder
13. Baking Soda
14. Ball Real Fruit Instant Pectin
15. Bean Flour
16. Better Batter
17. Betterbody Foods Cacao Powder
18. Betterbody Foods Coconut MCT Oil: The Only Ingredient Is Coconut Oil
19. Bisquick Gluten Free Pancake & Waffle Mix
20. Bobs Red Mill 1-To-1 Baking Flour
21. Bobs Red Mill Gluten Free All Purpose Flour
22. Bobs Red Mill Egg Replacer
23. Brown Rice Flour
24. Brown Sugar
25. Buckwheat Flour
26. Canola Oil
27. Cassava Flour
28. Certo Pectin
29. Chia Seeds
30. Chi-Chi's Sweet Corn Cake Mix

A COMPREHENSIVE GLUTEN & DAIRY FREE GROCERY LIST

31. Chickpea Flour
32. Coconut Flakes
33. Coconut Flour
34. Coconut Milk (Can)
35. Coconut Oil
36. Coconut Sugar
37. Cocao Powder
38. Cocoa, Unsweetened
39. Corn Masa Flour
40. Corn Oil
41. Corn Starch
42. Corn Syrup
43. Cornmeal, White And Yellow
44. Crisco All Vegetable Shortening (Soybean Oil)
45. Cup4cup Gluten Free Flour Blend
46. Distilled White Vinegar
47. Dried Fruit
48. Edible Metallic Shimmer Spray
49. Energ Egg Replacer
50. Fava Bean Flour
51. Flax Seed
52. Fleischmanns Active Dry Yeast
53. Guar Gum, A Thickening Agent
54. Gelatin, Unflavored
55. Gerbs Dark Chocolate Chips
56. Ghirardelli Unsweetened Chocolate 70%, 100% Cacao Baking Bar
57. Grapeseed Oil
58. Hershey's Cocoa
59. Holland House Cooking Wine Sherry
60. Katz White Bread Mix
61. Karo Corn Syrup
62. Kikkoman Panko Gluten Free
63. King Arthur Gluten Free All Purpose Baking Mix
64. Lard
65. Lodi Unbaked All-Purpose Lupin Flour
66. Millet Flour
67. Namaste Brown Rice Flour
68. Namaste Gluten Free Italian Herb Coating Mix
69. Namaste Millet Flour
70. Namaste Gluten Free Pizza Crust Mix

A COMPREHENSIVE GLUTEN & DAIRY FREE GROCERY LIST

71. Namaste Quinoa Flour
72. Namaste Sorghum Flour
73. Namaste Tapioca Starch
74. Namaste Xanthan Gum
75. Natures Earthly Choice Goji Berry Powder
76. Nature's Earthly Choice All Natural Nut Flour Blend
77. Non-Stick Cooking Spray (*Except* Bakers Joy With Flour)
78. Nutritional Yeast Flakes
79. Nuts And Seeds, Unseasoned Plain
80. Oat Flour
81. Olive Oil
82. Oregon Specialty Fruit All Natural Whole Pitted Red Tart Cherries In Water
83. Orgran Gluten Free Self-Raising Flour
84. Pam Olive Oil Cooking Spray
85. Pamela's All Purpose Gluten Free Flour
86. Peanut Oil
87. Pillsbury Gluten Free Flour
88. Potato Starch
89. Powdered Sugar
90. Private Selection Mediterranean Garlic Dipping Oil
91. Psyllium Husk
92. Quinoa Flour
93. Red Palm Oil (Nutiva Is One Brand To Look For)
94. Red Star All Natural Active Dry Yeast (Not Brewer's Yeast)
95. Red Star Quick Rise Instant Yeast
96. Safflower Oil
97. Schar Gluten Free Bread Crumbs
98. Scharffen Berger Unsweetened Natural Cocoa Powder
99. Sorghum
100. Sunflower Oil
101. Sure-Jell Original Premium Fruit Pectin (All Pectin, Any Brand)
102. Tapioca Flour
103. Tapioca Starch
104. Teff Flour
105. Vegetable Oil (Which Is Soybean Oil)
106. Walnut Oil
107. White Granulated Sugar
108. Xanthan Gum
109. Yeast, Baker's Yeast & Active Dry Yeast

A COMPREHENSIVE GLUTEN & DAIRY FREE GROCERY LIST

BEVERAGES

1. 7Up And Diet 7up
2. All Water Like Plain, Carbonated, Sparkling, Flavored.
3. Almond Milk (Check Your Refrigerated Section For Silk, Blue Diamond & Others)
4. Apple Cider
5. Apple Juice
6. Arizona Fruit Punch
7. Arizona Green Tea
8. Bai Beverages
9. Bodyarmor Fruit Punch Super Drink
10. Bolthouse Farms Berry Boost Fruit Juice Smoothie
11. Bolthouse Farms Plant Milk
12. Bolthouse Farms Strawberry Banana Fruit Smoothie
13. Bragg Apple Cider Vinegar Ginger Spice Drink
14. Calamatta Juice
15. Capri Sun
16. Cherry Bay Orchards 100% Tart Cherry Juice
17. Clamato Tomato Cocktail
18. Coconut Milk
19. Coconut Water
20. Coca-Cola And Diet Coke
21. Coffee
22. Core Hydration Perfect Ph Water
23. Country Time Lemonade Flavored Drink Mix
24. Cranberry Juice
25. Crystal Light Drink Mix
26. Dr. Pepper
27. Faraon Aloe Vera Juice
28. Flaxmilk
29. Gatorade
30. Ginger Ale
31. Goodbelly Probiotics Juice Drinks
32. Grape Juice
33. Grapefruit Juice
34. Hawaiian Punch

A COMPREHENSIVE GLUTEN & DAIRY FREE GROCERY LIST

35. Hi-C Punch
36. Juice
37. Jumex Mango Nectar
38. Kern's Guava Nectar
39. Kern's Mango Nectar
40. Kevita Cleansing Probiotic Apple Cider Vinegar Tonic, Turmeric Ginger
41. Kevita Lemon Cayenne Sparkling Probiotic Drink
42. Kevita Master Brew Kombucha Tart Cherry
43. Kevita Sparkling Probiotic Drink, Lemon Ginger
44. Kevita Sparkling Probiotic Mojita Lime Mint Coconut Drink
45. Kevita Strawberry Acai Coconut Sparkling Probiotic Drink
46. Kool-Aid
47. Lemon Juice
48. Lemonade
49. Lime Juice
50. Lipton Green Tea Citrus
51. Lipton Iced Tea Mix
52. Lipton Iced Tea Peach
53. Martinelli's Gold Medal Sparkling Cider
54. Minute Maid Fruit Punch
55. Minute Maid Peach Fruit Juice
56. Mio Liquid Flavored Water Enhancer
57. Mountain Dew
58. Monster Energy Drink
59. Naked Blue Machine Juice Smoothie
60. Naked Mighty Mango Juice Smoothie, But...
    i. Naked Green Machine Has Wheat (A Gluten)
    ii. Naked Protein & Greens Juice Has Dairy
    iii. Naked Protein Zone Juice Smoothie Has Whey, (A Dairy Ingredient)
61. Naked Red Machine Juice Smoothie
62. Naked Strawberry & Banana Juice Smoothie
63. Odwalla Mango Tango 100% Juice Smoothie
64. Odwalla Original Superfood 100% Juice Smoothie
65. Orange Juice
66. Pacific Organic Almond Non-Dairy Beverage (Shelf Stable Box)
67. Pacific Organic Coconut Non Dairy Beverage (Shelf Stable Box)
68. Pepsi And Diet Pepsi
69. Perrier
70. Pineapple Juice

A COMPREHENSIVE GLUTEN & DAIRY FREE GROCERY LIST

71. Pomegranate Juice
72. Powerade Sports Drink
73. Prune Juice
74. Red Bull
75. Rice Milk
76. Simply Fruit Punch Juice Drink
77. Simply Lemonade
78. Simply Smoothie's, All Flavors
79. Snapple
80. Soft Drinks; All Soft Drinks And All Diet Soft Drinks
81. Soy Milk (A Soy Product)
82. Sparkling Ice Brand Sparkling Water
83. Sparkling Water
84. Sprite
85. Starbucks Blonde Roast Iced Coffee (In-Store)
86. Sunny D
87. Tang Orange Powdered Drink Mix
88. Tea
89. Tequila
90. Tomato Juice
91. Torani Sugar Free Flavoring Syrup
92. Trader Joe's Almond Cashew & Macadamia Nut Beverage
93. Trader Joe's Almond Nog
94. Tropicana Essentials Probiotics Strawberry Banana Juice
95. V-8 Splash Berry Blend
96. V-8 Splash Tropical Blend
97. V-8 Vegetable Juice
98. Vitamin Water
99. Water
100. Welch's Red Grape Sparkling Juice Cocktail

A COMPREHENSIVE GLUTEN & DAIRY FREE GROCERY LIST

BREAD

1. Against The Grain: Cinnamon Raisin Bagels
2. Against The Grain: Gourmet Vermont Country Rolls (Be Aware Not All "Against The Grain" Breads Are Dairy Free.
3. All But Gluten Sliced Bread
4. Amy's Organic Sandwich Rounds, Boxed In The Frozen Foods Dept. (Use As Little Pizza Crust)
5. Bfree Wheat And Gluten Free Bread
6. Bobs Red Mill Gluten Free Biscuit & Baking Mix
7. Bobs Red Mill Gluten Free Cinnamon Raisin Bread Mix
8. Bfree Gluten Free Sandwich Bread
9. Cali'flour Foods Gluten Free Low Carb Artisan Style Pizza Crustcanyon Bakehouse Gluten Free Bread
10. Ener-G Foods Tapioca Hot Dog Buns
11. Ener-G Foods Yeast Free Brown Rice Loaf
12. Ener-G Foods Tapioca Loaf Classic White
13. Ener-G Foods Multigrain Brown Rice Loaf
14. Food For Life Gluten Free Bread
15. Food For Life Brown Rice Gluten Free Tortillas
16. Franz Gluten Free Bread
17. Glutino' Gluten Free English Muffins
18. Julian Bakery Ketothin Pizza Crust Mix
19. La Banderita Corn Tortillas (Possible Cross Contamination)
20. Livegfree Bread
21. Livegfree Plain Tortilla Wraps
22. Katz Gluten Free English Muffins
23. Kinnikinnick Gf White Soft Sandwich Bread

24. Kinnikinnick Gluten Free English Muffins
25. Mina's Purely Divine Gluten Free Bread Mix
26. Mission Gluten Free Tortilla
27. Mission White Corn Tortillas
28. Namaste Foods Gluten Free Pizza Crust
29. Pamela's Gluten Free Bread Mix
30. Rudi's Gluten Free Original Sandwich Bread
31. Sam's Choice Gluten Free Bread
32. Schar Gluten Free Ciabatta Bread
33. Schar Gluten Free Bread, Rolls, And Buns
34. Schar Gluten Free Italian (Crunchy) Breadsticks
35. Simple Mills Artisan Bread Almond Flour Mix, Box
36. Simple Truth Fresh Gluten Free Pizza Crust Mix
37. Three Bakers Gluten Free 7 Ancient Grain Bread
38. Toufayan Tortilla Wraps, Gluten Free
39. Trader Joe's Gluten Free White Sandwich Bread
40. Udi's Gluten Free French Baguettes
41. Udi's Gluten Free Bagels
42. Udi's Gluten Free Bread (Often Found In The Freezer Section)
43. Udi's Gluten Free Blueberry Muffins (Premade)
44. Udi's Gluten Free Hamburger Buns
45. Udi's Gluten Free Hot Dog Buns
46. Udi's Gluten Free Tortillas (Many Of The Udi Brand Products Will Be Found In The Freezer Section Of You Grocery Store.)

BOXED MIXES, ICING & PIE

> *The ingredient, "cocoa butter" is dairy free. It is actually the oil from the cocoa bean.*

1. Betty Crocker Chocolate Gluten Free Brownie Mix
2. Bobs Red Mill Gluten Free Chocolate Chip Cookie Mix
3. D'Gari Flan
4. Food Coloring
5. Glutino Gluten Free Pantry, Double Chocolate Brownie Mix
6. Godiva Chocolate Instant Pudding Mix
7. Godiva White Chocolate Vanilla Bean Instant Pudding Mix
8. Great Value Cookie Icing, 7 Ounce
9. Great Value Decorating Cupcake Icing, 8.4oz
10. Great Value Decorating Icing, 4.25 Ounce Tube
11. Great Value Gluten Free Brownie Mix
12. Great Value Unflavored Gelatin
13. Hershey's Instant Pudding Mix
14. Immaculate Gluten Free Classic Sugar Cookie Mix
15. Jello
16. Jello Banana Cream Pudding Pie Filling
17. Jello Lemon Pudding Pie Filling
18. Jello Tapioca Fat Free Cook Serve Pudding Pie Filling Mix
19. Jello Vanilla Instant Pudding (In The Box That You Make Using Dairy Free Milk)
20. Jolly Rancher Gelatin

A COMPREHENSIVE GLUTEN & DAIRY FREE GROCERY LIST

21. King Arthur Gluten Free Chocolate Cake Mix
22. Kinnikinnick Gluten Free Angel Food Cake Mix
23. Knox Gelatin
24. Marshmallow Creme
25. Marshmallows
26. Mi-Del Gluten Free Pie Crust, Graham Style (For Those Of You That Are Sensitive To Cross Contamination Please Note That Per The Company This Product Is Processed In A Plant That Processes Milk, Nut And Soy Products)
27. Namaste Foods Gluten Free Chocolate Cake Mix
28. Namaste Foods Gluten Free Spice Cake Mix
29. Pamela's Gluten Free Vanilla Cake Mix
30. Pie Filling (Most Brands)
31. Pillsbury Creamy Supreme Coconut Pecan Frosting
32. Pillsbury Frost Vanilla Marshmallow Fluffy Frosting
33. Royal Delights Pie Filling Mix Key Lime Crème (Per The Company's Web Site This Is Gluten Free)
34. Royal Delights Salted Caramel Dessert Mix
35. Royal Delights White Chocolate Dessert Mix
36. Simple Mills Organic Chocolate Frosting With Coconut Oil
37. Simple Mills Organic Vanilla **Frosting** With Coconut Oil
38. Simple Mills Vanilla Cupcake Mix
39. Sprinkles (Most Brands)
40. Tapioca (Ex: Kraft Minute Tapioca)
41. Udi's Brownie Mug Cake

MONONITRATE {VITAMIND B1}, RIBOFLAVIN {VITAMIN B2, FOLIC ACID} SOYBEAN OIL, SUGAR, PARTIALLY HYDROGENATED COTTONSEED OIL, SALT, LEAVENING (BAKING SODA AND/OR CALCIUM PHOSPHATE), HIGH FRUCTOSE CORN SYRUP, SOY LECITHIN, MALTED BARLEY FLOUR, NATURAL FLAVOR.
CONTAINS WHEAT, SOY.

Don't rely on the front of the packaging to tell you if a product contains gluten or dairy.

Many products place a small statement on the back of the packaging near the bottom usually. Often you can find it just below the ingredient list.

BREAKFAST

1. Amy's Breakfast Scramble (With Tofu)
2. Applegate Naturals Chicken & Apple Breakfast Sausage Patties
3. Applegate Naturals Chicken & Maple Breakfast Sausage
4. Applegate Naturals Chicken & Sage Breakfast Sausage
5. Applegate Naturals Classic Pork Breakfast Sausage
6. Applegate Naturals Bacon And Turkey Bacon
7. Birch Benders Paleo Pancake & Waffle Mix
8. Cereal (See The Chapter On CEREAL)
9. Enjoy Life Soft Baked Breakfast Fruit & Oat Oval Breakfast Bars
10. Jennie-O All Natural Turkey Sausage (Roll)
11. Jennie-O Turkey Bacon
12. Gluten Free Waffles: Check The Chapter On Frozen Foods
13. Glutenull Quinoa Granola
14. Great Value Grape Jelly
15. Hormel Black Label Bacon
16. Kashi Chew Nut Butter Bars GF
17. Katz Gluten Free Cinnamon Raisin English Muffins
18. Katz Gluten Free Cinnamon Rugelech (Cinnamon Rolls)
19. Katz Gluten Free Glazed Donuts
20. Kinnikinnick Quinoa Spice Muffins (In The Frozen Section)
21. Libre Naturals Gluten Free Oatmeal
22. Maple Syrup
23. Martha White Gluten Free Blueberry Muffin Mix
24. Molasses
25. Namaste Foods Gluten Free Waffle & Pancake Mix
26. Oats Overnight
27. Orgran Stonemilled Buckwheat Pancake Mix
28. Pamela's Pancake & Waffle Mix, Glutenfree, Non-Dairy (Possible Cross Contamination From Dairy)
29. Sam's Choice Uncured Turkey Bacon
30. Simple Mills Almond Flour Pancake Mix
31. Sunfood Superfoods Organic Acai Maqui Bowl Powder
32. Syrup??
33. Welch's Concord Grape Jelly

A COMPREHENSIVE GLUTEN & DAIRY FREE GROCERY LIST

CEREAL

As with every chapter: Some products are gluten free but not dairy free, and vice-versa. Only products that are both gluten and dairy free are included in this list.

1. Apple Cinnamon Cheerios Gluten Free
2. Arrowhead Mills Gluten Free Maple Buckwheat Flakes
3. Bakery On Main Oatmeal
4. Bear Naked Granola Bites Peanut Butter & Honey
5. Bear Naked Granola V'nilla Almond
6. Bobs Red Mill Gluten Free Muesli
7. Bobs Red Mill Gluten Free Oats
8. Cheerios Gluten Free
9. Chocolate Cheerios Gluten Free
10. Chocolate Chex Gluten Free
11. Cinnamon Chex Gluten Free Cereal
12. Cocoa Pebbles Gluten Free
13. Corn Chex, Gluten Free
14. Frosted Cheerios, Gluten Free
15. Honey Nut Gluten Free Chex Cereal
16. Julian Bakery Progranola
17. Kashi Organic Indigo Morning
18. Katz Gluten Free Farfel
19. Kix Cereals: All Varieties
20. Lucky Charms Gluten Free
21. Malt-O-Meal Gluten Free Cocoa Dyno-Bites, Bag
22. Malt-O-Meal Gluten Free Crispy Rice, Bag
23. Malt-O-Meal Gluten Free Fruity Dyno Bites, Bag
24. Maple Cheerios, Gluten Free
25. Multi Grain Cheerios Gluten Free Cereal
26. Nature's Path Organic Mesa Sunrise
27. Post Fruity Pebbles, Gluten Free
28. Quaker Gluten Free Instant Oatmeal
29. Quaker Gluten Free Oats
30. Rice Chex
31. Trader Joe's Crispy Quinoa Stars Cereal
32. Trader Joe's Neapolitan Puffs Cereal
33. Udi's Au Naturel Granola
34. Very Berry Cheerios, Gluten Free

CANNED FOODS

Canned and Dried Beans

1. Adzuki Beans
2. Amy's Vegetarian Organic Baked Beans
3. Anasazi Beans
4. Black Beans
5. Black Eyed Peas
6. Bushes Best Original Baked Beans
7. Butter Beans
8. Cannellini Beans
9. Chick Peas
10. Eden Organic Black Soy Beans
11. Fava Beans
12. Garbanzo Beans
13. Green Beans
14. Green Peas
15. Kidney Beans
16. Kroger Black Beans
17. Lentils (By Themselves)
18. Libby's Green Beans
19. Lima Beans
20. Peas
21. Pinto Beans
22. Mung Beans
23. Navy Beans
24. Northern Beans
25. Old El Paso Refried Beans
26. Pacific Organic Baked Beans Vegetarian
27. Pacific Organic Refried Black Beans With Green Chiles
28. Red Beans
29. Refried Beans: Similar To The Ingredients On Rosarita Refried Beans Which Are Gluten And Dairy Free.
30. Runner Beans
31. Split Peas
32. Wax Beans

A COMPREHENSIVE GLUTEN & DAIRY FREE GROCERY LIST

Canned and Packaged Meats/Seafoods

1. Abalone
2. Anchovies
3. Armour Corned Beef, Canned
4. Armour Potted Meat
5. Big Johns Red Hots Pickled Sausage
6. Bumble Bee Clams
7. Bumble Bee Chipotle Seasoned Tuna Fish Pouch
8. Bubble Bee Pink Salmon
9. Bubble Bee Sardines
10. Canned Tuna, Salmon, Mackeral, Sardines, Etc
11. Canned Ham
12. Caviar
13. Chicken Of The Sea Sardines And Sardines In Mustard Sauce
14. Clams
15. Deming's Red Sockeye Salmon
16. Deviled Ham Spread
17. El Mexicano Sliced Pickled Carrots
18. Hormel Corned Beef, Canned
19. Hormel Beef Tamales In Chili Sauce: All Of The Ingredients Listed Are Gluten And Dairy Free
20. Keystone Chicken, Canned
21. Keystone Ground Beef, Canned
22. Keystone Pork, Canned
23. Keystone Turkey, Canned
24. Libby's Vienna Sausage, Canned
25. Mackerel
26. Oysters
27. Pampa Giant Calamari In Garlic Sauce
28. Pickled Cured Pork Hocks
29. Pigs Feet
30. Polar Smoked Peppered Herring Fillets
31. Salmon
32. Shrimp
33. Spam With Chorizo
34. Spam, Classic
35. Spam Oven Roasted Turkey

36. Spam Singles Classic
37. Spam Spread
38. Swanson Canned Chicken
39. Trans Ocean Crab Classic Flake Style Imitation Crab
40. Tuna
41. Tushonka Canned Stewed Mutton Chunks, Canned
42. Valley Fresh 100% Natural Chicken Breast In Water (Canned)

Canned and Packaged Vegetables

1. Artichokes
2. Asparagus
3. Baby Corn
4. Bamboo Shoots
5. Beets
6. Carrots
7. Chile's
8. Collard Greens
9. Corn
10. Garlic
11. Green Beans
12. Hearts Of Palm
13. Hominy
14. Lima Beans
15. Sauerkraut
16. Mushrooms
17. Mustard Greens
18. Jarred Pearl Onions
19. Okra
20. Peas
21. Peppers
22. Pickled Okra
23. Pumpkin
24. Spinach
25. String Beans
26. Sweet Potato
27. Tomatoes
28. Turnip Greens
29. Water Chestnuts
30. Wax Beans
31. Yams
32. Zucchini And Squash

Canned and Packaged Fruits

1. Applesauce
2. Canned And Jarred Fruit
3. Cranberry Sauce
4. Del Monte Fruit Cups
5. Dried Fruit Should Be Gluten And Dairy Free. Check The Label. An Example Of A Gluten And Dairy Free Dried Fruit Is Sunsweet Apricots, Pitted Dates, And Prunes.
6. Dole Cherry Mixed Fruit Cups
7. Dole Fruit Bowls
8. Dole Mandarin Oranges
9. Dole Pineapple Chunks
10. Dole Tropical Fruit
11. Maraschino Cherries, Jar
12. Raisins

Canned Other

1. Amore Tomato Paste
2. California Sun-Dry Sun Dried Tomatoes
3. Capers
4. Cento Tomato Paste
5. Contadina Tomato Paste
6. Corned Beef Hash (If You Have A Reaction To Corned Beef Hash It Could Be From Cross Contamination)
7. Hatch Gluten Free Diced Green Chiles
8. Kimchi
9. Kroger Sloppy Joe Sandwich Sauce
10. La Victoria Diced Green Chiles
11. Manwich Has No Ingredients That Contain Gluten. If This Product Bothers You It May Be Caused By Cross Contamination.
12. Olives
13. Ortega Diced Green Chiles
14. Thai Kitchen Unsweetened Coconut Milk

CONDIMENTS

BARBECUE SAUCE

1. Bone Suckin' Sauce
2. G. Hughes Smokehouse Sugar Free Bbq Sauce
3. Great Value Tomato Ketchup
4. Guy Fieri Barbeque Sauce
5. Heinz Tomato Ketchup
6. Hunts Tomato Ketchup
7. Kc Masterpiece Original Barbecue Sauce
8. Kinder's Roasted Garlic Bbq Sauce
9. Kroger Original Tomato Ketchup
10. Sweet Baby Ray's Barbecue Sauce

Dressing

1. Annie's Balsamic Vinaigrette Dressing
2. Apple Cider Vinegar
3. Balsamic Vinegar
4. Bragg Organic Apple Cider Vinaigrette Dressing
5. Brianna's Honey Dijon Mustard Dressing
6. Daiya Blue Cheese Dressing
7. Daiya Caesar Dressing
8. Daiya Homestyle Ranch Dressing
9. Distilled White Vinegar
10. Girard's Light Champagne Dressing
11. Great Value Real Mayonnaise
12. Ken's Steak House Honey Mustard Dressing
13. Ken's Steak House Simply Vinaigrette Olive Oil & Vinegar
14. Kraft Catalina Dressing
15. Kraft Mayonnaise With Olive Oil
16. Kraft Real Mayo
17. Kraft Reduced Fat Mayonnaise With Olive Oil
18. Kroger Olive Oil Mayo
19. Marzetti Simply Dressed Vinaigrette Balsamic
20. Marzetti Sweet & Sour Dressing
21. Marzetti Country French Dressing

A COMPREHENSIVE GLUTEN & DAIRY FREE GROCERY LIST

22. Miracle Whip Salad Dressing
23. Oil: All Oil
24. Organicville Non-Dairy Ranch Dressing
25. Organicville Non-Dairy Thousand Island Dressing
26. Primal Kitchen Mayo Avocado Oil
27. Primal Kitchen Ranch, Greek Or Honey Mustard Dressing
28. Private Selection Orange Poppy Seed Dressing
29. Sesame Oil
30. Simple Truth Organic Rosemary Honey Mustard
31. Simply Organic Garlic Vinaigrette Dressing Mix Packet
32. Simply Organic Italian Dressing Mix Packet
33. Sir Kensington's Avocado Oil Mayonnaise
34. Vinegar: All Vinegar *Except* Malt Vinegar.
35. Walden Farms Asian Calorie Free Dressing
36. Walden Farms Bacon Ranch Calorie Free Dressing
37. Walden Farms Blue Cheese Dressing
38. Walden Farms Caesar Calorie Free Dressing
39. Walden Farms Calorie Free Balsamic Vinaigrette Dressing
40. Walden Farms Chipotle Ranch Dressing
41. Walden Farms Creamy Bacon Dressing
42. Walden Farms French Calorie Free Dressing
43. Walden Farms Honey Balsamic Vinaigrette Dressing
44. Walden Farms Honey Dijon Calorie Free Dressing
45. Walden Farms Italian Calorie Free Dressing
46. Walden Farms Italian With Sundried Tomato Dressing
47. Walden Farms Pear & White Balsamic Vinaigrette Dressing
48. Walden Farms Raspberry Vinaigrette Dressing
49. Walden Farms Russian Dressing
50. Walden Farms Sesame Ginger Dressing
51. Walden Farms Sweet Onion Dressing
52. Walden Farms Thousand Island Dressing
53. Wegmans Cilantro Lime Marinade
54. Wegmans Lemon & Garlic Marinade
55. Wegmans Rosemary Balsamic Marinade For Lamb Or Chicken

MISCELLANEOUS

1. A-1 Steak Sauce: If You Have A Reaction It May Be From Cross-Contamination
2. Boar's Head Honey Mustard
3. Bragg Liquid Aminos All Purpose Seasoning
4. Bragg Premium Nutritional Yeast Seasoning
5. Chi-Chi's Taco Sauce
6. Dales Steak Seasoning Liquid
7. Famous Dave's Signature Spicy Pickle Relish
8. Follow Your Heart Vegan Honey Mustard Dressing
9. Frank's Redhot Buffalo Wings Sauce
10. French's Classic Yellow Mustard
11. French's Honey Mustard
12. French's Worcestershire Sauce
13. Golden Farms Vidalia Onion Steak Sauce
14. Gopal's Rawmesan Parmesan Cheese Alternative
15. Grey Poupon Dijon Mustard
16. Great Value Dijon Mustard
17. Great Value Real Bacon Pieces
18. Great Value Worcestershire Sauce
19. Great Value Yellow Mustard
20. Heinz Sweet Relish
21. Hormel Real Bacon Bits
22. Horseradish
23. Hot Sauces: Most Hot Sauce Will Be Gluten Free. Check Your Labels.
24. Inglehoffer Stone Ground Mustard
25. Kroger Honey Mustard
26. Kroger Real Bacon Bits
27. Kroger Spicy Brown Mustard
28. Kroger Sweet Relish
29. Kroger Yellow Mustard
30. Lea & Perrins Original Worcestershire Sauce
31. Lee Kum Kee Gluten Free Panda Brand Oyser Sauce
32. Mayonnaise
33. Minced Garlic, Jar
34. Mt Olive Sweet Relish
35. Mustard
36. Nooch It! Organic Dairy Free Cashew Grated Cheeze

A COMPREHENSIVE GLUTEN & DAIRY FREE GROCERY LIST

37. Pbfit Plus Vegan Organic Plant Protein
38. Pickles
39. Salsa: Most Salsa Will Be Gluten Free But Check Your Label
40. Sesame Oil
41. Simple Truth Organic Smoky Chipotle Pepper Hot Sauce
42. Sky Valley Gluten Free Sriracha Sauce
43. Stubbs Beef Marinade
44. Sweet Baby Ray's Honey Mustard Dipping Sauce
45. Sweet Baby Ray's Sweet 'N Sour Sauce
46. Tabasco
47. Tahini
48. Tamarind
49. Vlasic Dill Relish
50. Wrights All Natural Liquid Smoke

SALSA

1. Amy's Salsa Chipotle
2. Chi-Chi's Salsa
3. Dei Fratelli Salsa
4. Herdez Guacamole Salsa
5. Herdez Roasted Salsa Verde
6. La Victoria Fire Roasted Diced Jalapeños Hot (Diced, Whole)
7. La Victoria Fire Roasted Green Chiles (Diced, Whole)
8. La Victoria Green Enchilada Sauce
9. La Victoria Nacho Sliced Jalapeños
10. La Victoria Red Enchilada Sauce La Victoria Salsa Cilantro
11. La Victoria Suprema Salsa La Victoria Thick & Chunky Salsa
12. La Victoria Thick N' Chunk Salsa Verde
13. Pace Salsa
14. **Salsa In General Is Gluten And Dairy Free But Check Your Label**.
15. Taco Bell Fire Sauce
16. Trader Joe's Roasted Salsa

SOY SAUCE & OTHER ASIAN SAUCES

1. Coconut Aminos
2. Huy Fong Foods Sambal Oelek Ground Fresh Chili Paste (Jar)
3. Kikkoman Gluten Free Soy Sauce
4. Kikkoman Gluten Free Teriyaki Sauce
5. La Choy Stir Fry Sauce, Original
6. Simple Truth Organic Sesame Teriyaki Marinade
7. Tamari

VINEGAR

1. Apple Cider Vinegar
2. Balsamic Vinegar
3. Distilled White Vinegar
4. Red Wine Vinegar
5. Rice Vinegar
6. White Wine Vinegar
   Basically All Vinegar With The Exception Of Malt Vinegar

A COMPREHENSIVE GLUTEN & DAIRY FREE GROCERY LIST

FRUIT: PRODUCE

Frozen, fresh, canned, dried: so long as it is the only ingredient with the exception of a sweetener perhaps. Check your labels to be sure. Keep it simple.

1. Apples
2. Apricot
3. Banana
4. Berries
5. Blueberries
6. Blackberries
7. Cantaloupe
8. Carob
9. Casaba Melon
10. Cherries
11. Coconut
12. Currants
13. Cranberries
14. Dates
15. Dragon Fruit
16. Fig
17. Grapefruit
18. Grapes
19. Guava
20. Honeydew
21. Kiwi
22. Kumquat
23. Lemons
24. Limes
25. Lychee
26. Mandarin Oranges
27. Mango
28. Melon
29. Nectarines
30. Oranges
31. Papaya
32. Peaches
33. Pears
34. Persimmon

35. Pineapple (Not Difficult To Slice Up With A Knife! Give It A Try)
36. Plantain
37. Plum
38. Pomegranate
39. Raspberries
40. Rhubarb
41. Star Fruit
42. Strawberries
43. Tangerine
44. Watermelon

FROZEN FOODS

All vegetables that do not have sauce or seasonings
All fruits that do not have anything added

BREAD
Many brands of gluten free bread are found in the frozen foods section of your grocery store.

BREAKFAST

Be sure to also check the breakfast chapter for more breakfast foods.

1. Amy's Brand Has Several Breakfast Burritos And Scrambles That Are Both Gluten And Dairy Free. But Not All. They Do Label Their Products Well.
2. Kashi Gluten Free Waffles GF
3. Kinnikinnick Muffins
4. Natures Path Organic Gluten Free Waffles
5. Vans Gluten Free Blueberry Waffles
6. Vans Gluten Free Original Waffles

DESSERTS

1. Daiya New York Cheezecake (Dairy Free, Gluten Free, Soy Free)
2. Great Value Strawberry Fruit Bars
3. Haagen-Dazs Non-Dairy Coconut Caramel Frozen Dessert
4. Halo Top Dairy Free Frozen Dessert
5. Icee Mix It Up Frozen Fruit Bars
6. Italian Ice
7. Kroger Freezer Pops
8. Luigi's Real Italian Ice
9. Otter Pops
10. Outshine Fruit Bars (Frozen Pops)
11. Popsicle Firecracker
12. Popsicle Ice Pops
13. Popsicle Jolly Rancher Flavored Pops
14. Sherbet: Don't Assume Sherbet Is Dairy Free! Most Have Milk And Skim Milk
15. Simple Truth Organic Dairy Free Frozen Fruit Bars
16. So Delicious Dairy Free Coconut Milk Gluten Free Non-Dairy Frozen
17. Talenti Dairy-Free Sorbetto

[Ben & Jerry's has a non-dairy ice cream but it has gluten. On the ingredient list of the Peanut Butter flavored frozen dessert "wheat flour" is listed. Ben & Jerry's also has soy.

ENTREES

1. Amy's Bowls, Baked Ziti
2. Amy's Bowls, Brown Rice, Black-Eyed Peas And Veggies
3. Amy's Bowls Brown Rice & Vegetables
4. Amy's Bowls, Harvest Casserole (This Includes Tofu)
5. Amy's Bowls, Paella
6. Amy's Bowls Sweet & Sour Rice And Tofu
7. Amy's Bowls Teriyaki
8. Amy's Chinese Noodles & Veggies In Cashew Cream Sauce
9. Amy's Vegan Cheeze & Black Bean Enchilada
10. Amy's Gluten Free Dairy Free Rice Mac & Cheeze
11. Amy's Gluten Free Non-Dairy Black Bean Vegetable Enchilada
12. Amy's Gluten Free Non Dairy Organic Beans & Rice Burrito
13. Amy's Gluten And Dairy Free Vegetable Lasagna
14. Amy's Light & Lean Quinoa & Black Beans With Butternut Squash And Chard
15. Amy's Indian Vegetable Korma
16. Amy's Non-Dairy Rice Macaroni And Cheeze
17. Amy's Thai Pad Thai
18. Applegate Naturals Gluten Free Chicken Nuggets
19. Beetnik Organic Chicken Chili Verde
20. Beetnik Organic Lemongrass Chicken With Green Beans
21. Beetnik Organic Moroccan Inspired Chicken Stew
22. Beetnik Sesame Ginger Chicken With Broccoli, Zucchini, Carrots, Bell Peppers, Spices And Rice
23. Blake's Gluten Free Chicken Pot Pie
24. Blakes Gluten Free Shepherd's Pie
25. Golden Platter All Natural Chicken Tenders
26. Golden Platter Dino Nuggets
27. Golden Platter Disney Winnie The Pooh Honey Nuggets
28. Great Value Chicken And Coconut Curry, Whole30 Meal
29. Great Value Mediterranean Inspired Chicken Whole30 Meal
30. Great Value Spinach Pesto Chicken & Vegetables, Whole30 Meal
31. Great Value Roasted Orange Chicken & Vegetables Whole30 Meal
32. Great Value Rosemary Chicken & Vegetables, Whole30 Meal

33. Healthy Choice Cajun Style Chicken & Shrimp (This Is The Only Healthy Choice Entrée I Could Find That Was Both Gluten And Dairy Free At The Time Of My Research)
34. Lean Cuisine Marketplace Chicken With Almonds,
    - (Not All Of The Lean Cuisine Marketplace Frozen Dinners Are Gluten And Dairy Free.
    - I Have Listed All Approved Meals Here That I Could Find At The Time Of This Printing)
35. Lean Cuisine Marketplace Chicken With Almonds (Also Nightshade Free)
36. Lean Cuisine Marketplace Chicken Cashew Stir Fry
37. Lean Cuisine Marketplace Mango Chicken With Coconut Rice
38. Lean Cuisine Marketplace Sweet & Sour Chicken
39. Lean Cuisine Marketplace Sweet & Spicy Korean-Style Beef
40. Lean Cuisine Marketplace Sweet & Spicy Harissa Meatballs (Nightshade Alert)
41. Lean Cuisine Marketplace Sweet & Spicy Korean Style Beef
42. Lean Cuisine Origins Coconut Chickpea Curry
43. Lean Cuisine Pomegranate Chicken With Green Beans
44. Saffron Road Beef Bulgogi With Brown Rice

FRUITS

All frozen fruit is gluten and dairy free. Choose frozen fruit that has an ingredients list of just the fruit(s) and nothing else.

MISCELLANEOUS

1. Amy's Indian Curry Korma Wrap
2. Applegate Naturals Gluten Free Beef Corn Dogs
3. Beatnik Organic Chicken Meatballs In Resealable Bag (Frozen Foods)
4. Foster Farms Gluten Free Breast Nuggets
5. Foster Farms Gluten Free Chicken Breast Strips
6. Foster Farms Gluten Free Corn Dogs
7. Hilary's Eat Well Veggie Burger
8. Tofu (A Soy Product)
9. Wholly Wholesome Gluten Free Pie Shells

PIZZA

1. Amy's Gluten Free Dairy Free Rice Crust Pizza
2. Amy's Vegan Meatless Pepperoni
3. Amy's Roasted Vegetable Pizza, No Cheese (Gf)
4. Bold Organics Vegan Cheese Pizza With Gf Crust
5. Daiya Dairy Free Gluten Free Frozen Pizza
6. Kinnikinnick Gluten Free Personal Size Pizza Crusts
7. Manini's Gluten Free Pizza Crust
8. Sonoma Flatbreads Gluten Free Dairy Free Fire Roasted Vegetables Pizza

POTATOES

1. Frozen potatoes with potatoes as the only ingredient are most likely gluten free. Some companies have started to indicate on the label (check the back of the package) to state if the gluten free product was manufactured in a plant where there may be cross-contamination for those who are extremely sensitive.
2. Ore-Ida Golden Fries French Fried Potatoes
3. Ore-Ida Golden Tater Tots
4. Ore-Ida Shredded hash Brown Potatoes

VEGETABLES

All frozen vegetables, in and of themselves are gluten and dairy free. Choose frozen vegetables with an ingredients list of just the vegetable(s). No added ingredients like seasoning or sauce.

MEAT AND SEAFOOD DEPARTMENT

All meat and seafood that is not breaded or seasoned is gluten and dairy free.

1. Aidells Chicken & Apple Smoked Chicken Sausage
2. Al Fresco Sweet Apple Chicken Sausage
3. Amy's Sonoma Veggie Burger: Gluten Free, Dairy Free, Soy Free! It Does Have Potatoes (A Nightshade)
4. Applegate Bacon
5. Applegate Classic Pork Breakfast Sausage
6. Applegate Hot Dogs And Sausages
7. Applegate Naturals Gluten Free Chicken Tenders (Boxed)
8. Applegate Naturals Fajita Style Grilled Chicken Breast Strips, Boxed
9. Applegate Organic Turkey Burgers (Boxed)
10. Armour Bacon
11. Ball Park Franks
12. Bar S Hot Dogs
13. Bass
14. Beef
15. Beelers Bacon
16. Bluefish
17. Bob Evans Bacon
18. Boars Head Canadian Style Bacon
19. Boars Head Brand Smoked Imported Bacon
20. Boars Head Brand Hot Dogs
21. Bubba Burger (Gluten Free Hamburger Patties, Frozen)
22. Butterball Turkey Bacon
23. Carp
24. Catfish
25. Caviar
26. Chicken
27. Clams
28. Cod
29. Contessa Cutting Board Rockfish (Boxed)
30. Contessa Cutting Board Wild Salmon
31. Corned Beef
32. Crabs
33. Del Real Foods Shredded Chicken
34. Del Real Slow Cooked Pork Crnitas

A COMPREHENSIVE GLUTEN & DAIRY FREE GROCERY LIST

35. Farmland Bacon
36. Farmland Original Pork Sausage
37. Farmland Special Select Ham
38. Flounder
39. Frog Legs
40. Ground Beef
41. Ground Pork
42. Ground Turkey
43. Ground Chicken
44. Haddock
45. Halibut
46. Ham
47. Hormel Always Tender Fresh Meats
48. Hormel Cure 81 Diced Boneless Ham
49. Ian's Gluten Free Fish Sticks
50. Jennie-O Turkey Bratwurst
51. Jennie-O Ground Turkey
52. **Jennie-O Seasoned Turkey Burgers (Boxed)**
53. Jones Dairy Farm Canadian Bacon
54. Johnsonville Italian Sausage
55. Johnsonville Smoked Brats
56. Johnsonville Sweet Italian Sausage
57. Jolly Roger Fresh Pacific Oysters (Jar)
58. Kirkland Hot Dogs
59. Kirkland Signature Steak Strips (Boxed)
60. Lloyds Beef Brisket No Sauce
61. Lloyd's Pulled Pork, No Sauce
62. Lloyd's Ribs, All Varieties
63. Lloyd's Shredded Chicken With Bbq Sauce(Tub)
64. Lloyd's Shredded Beef In Original Bbq Sauce, (Tub)
65. Lobster
66. Mahi-Mahi
67. Mussels
68. Nathans Hot Dogs
69. Orange Roughy
70. Oscar Mayer Bacon
71. Oysters
72. Perch
73. Pier 33 Gourmet Langostino Lobster (Boxed)
74. Pike

75. Pollock
76. Pork
77. Pork Chops
78. Pork Roast
79. Pork Tenderloin
80. Red Snapper
81. Sardines
82. Scallops
83. Shrimp
84. Squid
85. Smithfield Pork Tenderloin
86. Sole
87. Talapia
88. Trans Ocean Crab Classic Imitation Crab
89. Trout
90. Tuna
91. Turkey
92. Veal
93. Wellshire Farms Hot Dogs And Products

MISCELLANEOUS

1. Corn Taco Shells: Likely To Be Gluten Free But Check The Label
2. Dynasty Gluten Free Rice Panko
3. Garden Of Eatin' Yellow Corn Taco Shells
4. Ian's Gluten Free Italian Panko Breadcrumbs
5. La Costena Pickled Jalapeno Nacho Slices
6. Live G Free Gluten Free French Fried Onions, Original
7. Kinnikinnick Graham Style Crumbs
8. OLD EL PASO TACO SHELLS
9. Ortega Yellow Corn Taco Shells
10. Raised Gluten Free Pumpkin Pie (Prepared Pie)
11. Simple Truth Organic Yellow Corn Taco Shells

NUTS AND SEEDS

1. Almonds
2. Bakers Angel Flake Coconut Sweetened
3. Bobs red mill coconut flakes
4. Brazil nuts
5. Cashews
6. Chestnuts
7. Chia seeds
8. Coconut, in and of itself is gluten and dairy free
9. Gefen Chestnuts Whole Shelled
10. Hazelnuts
11. Hemp seeds
12. Macadamia nuts
13. Peanuts
14. Pine nuts
15. Pistachio's
16. Pecans
17. Pumpkin seeds
18. Poppy seeds
19. Sesame seeds
20. Sunflower seeds
21. Walnuts

PACKAGED FOODS

1. 365 Almond Butter
2. Armour Real Bacon Bits
3. Betty Crocker 100% Real Mashed Potatoes
4. Banh Trang Viet Nam Rice Paper (Made With Tapioca)
5. Claussen Kosher Dill Pickles
6. Egg Roll Wraps: Look For One With Tapioca Or Coconut Flour. Example: Nuco Coconut Wraps
7. Great Value Instant Potatoes
8. Hershey's Milk Chocolate Syrup
9. Idaho Spuds Classic Mashed Potatoes
10. Idahoan Original Mashed Potatoes
11. Instant Potatoes Are Not All Gf And Df So Check The Ingredients List. For Example, Idahoan Buttery Homestyle Mashed Potatoes (Boxed) Have Nonfat Dry Milk Listed In The Ingredients List.
12. Katz Gluten Free Glazed Donut Holes
13. Maranatha Creamy Almond Butter
14. Old El Paso Stand 'N Stuff Taco Shells
15. Olives
16. Orgran Falafel Mix
17. Oscar Mayer Bacon Bits
18. Pbfit All Natural Peanut Butter Powder
19. Pearl Onions, Jarred
20. Pepperoncini
21. Pickled Eggs
22. Pickled Okra
23. Pickled Pigs Feet
24. Pickles
25. Utz Original Potato Stix

PASTA, GRAINS, RICE, BOXED POTATOES

1. Ancient harvest gluten free pasta
2. Barilla Gluten Free Pasta
3. Bobs Red Mill Gluten Free Corn Grits
4. Bobs Red Mill Whole Grain White Quinoa
5. Chia Seeds
6. Colavita Instant Polenta
7. Great Value Gluten Free Brown Rice Spaghetti, Penne, and elbow macaroni
8. Kroger gluten free spaghetti
9. La Choy Canned Chow Mein (per the co. the soy sauce is gluten free)
10. Lundberg organic gluten free spaghetti (brown rice pasta)
11. Lundberg Wild Blend Rice
12. Mahatma Yellow Saffron Rice Mix
13. Manischewitz Potato Pancake Mix (per the company, this is made in
    a. plant that processes wheat)
14. **Namaste gluten free Say Cheez macaroni & cheez dinner**
15. OrgraN Buckwheat Pasta
16. Rice is naturally gluten free but can sometimes be cross-contaminated
17. Ronzoni Gluten Free Pasta
18. Signature Select Gluten Free past
19. Simple truth organic gluten free penne
20. Thai Kitchen Stir Fry Rice Noodles
21. Uncle Ben's Ready Rice, Original
22. Quinoa

A COMPREHENSIVE GLUTEN & DAIRY FREE GROCERY LIST

REFRIGERATED

1. Almond Breeze Almond Milk Creamer
2. Califia Farms Cold Brew Coffee w/ almond milk
3. Chao Slices (cheese alternative)
4. Chobani non-dairy yogurt
5. Daiya dairy free cheese slices & shreds
6. Daiya dairy free cream cheese
7. Eggs
8. Follow Your Heart Parmesan Style Shredded Cheese Alternative
9. Food Merchants Traditional Italian Polenta
10. Kite hill dairy free cream cheese
11. Kroger Break-Free Liquid Egg Whites
12. Mocha mix original non-dairy coffee creamer
13. Non-dairy milks (see Beverages)
14. Nut Pods Unsweetened Dairy Free Creamer
15. Parma! Vegan Parmesan
16. Reddi-wip Non-Dairy made with Almond Milk Vegan Whipped Topping
17. Silk Dairy Free Yogurt (Soy Alert)
18. So delicious dairy free coconutmilk creamer
19. So Delicious Dairy Free Coconut Milk Yogurt
20. So delicious dairy free coco whip coconut whipped topping
21. Wholly Avocado Simply Avocado dip & spread (my favorite. The only ingredient is avocado so it is nightshade free!)
22. Wholly guacamole classic guacamole: avocados, vinegar, jalapeno peppers, salt, onion and garlic.

A COMPREHENSIVE GLUTEN & DAIRY FREE GROCERY LIST

DAIRY FREE BUTTER SUBSTITUTES

1. Country Crock Churn Style Vegetable Oil Spread
2. Earth Balance dairy free butter substitute
3. Ghee (for some. If it bothers you just omit it)
4. I Can't Believe It's Not Butter
5. Imperial Vegetable Oil Spread Butter Flavor
6. Nutiva Butter Flavored Coconut Oil
7. Pure blends avocado oil plant base butter
8. Pure blends coconut oil butter spread
9. Smart Balance Dairy Free butter substitute

LUNCHMEAT

1. Applegate Naturals brand
2. Applegate naturals genoa salami
3. Armour Meats
4. Bar S brand
5. Boars Head
6. Buddig Original
7. Butterball
8. Gallo Salame
9. Hormel Natural Choice lunchmeats
10. Jennie-O lunchmeats like turkey pastrami, turkey, turkey ham, etc
11. Land O'Frost
12. Oscar Mayer Deli Fresh

SHELF STABLE ENTREES

1. Hormel compleats chicken breast and gravy with mashed potatoes
2. Hormel Compleats Homestyle Beef Tips with mashed potatoes
3. Hormel compleats rice and chicken
4. Hormel compleats roast beef & gravy with mashed potatoes
5. Tasty Bite Thai Lime Rice (microwaveable packet)

A COMPREHENSIVE GLUTEN & DAIRY FREE GROCERY LIST

SNACK FOODS

1. 3-seed beet crackers
2. Absolutely gluten free classic coconut macaroons
3. Almond butter
4. Banana Chips
5. Brims Fired Pork Rinds
6. Cabo chips
7. Cashew butter
8. Cape Cod Blueberry Granola by GERBS (brand)
9. Chi-chi's chips are all gluten free. Check ingredients for dairy. Especially seasoned chips.
10. Chic Naturals Baked Crunchy Chickpea Snacks
11. Corn chips: so long as the ingredients are just corn, oil, salt. Some actually have the ingredient "whey" which is milk.
12. "*Food should taste good*" tortilla chips
13. Fritos original corn chips and Scoops
14. Fruit Roll-Ups
15. Garden of Eatin' baked blue tortilla chips
16. Glutino Gluten Free Snack Crackers, Sea Salt
17. Good Thins (Nabisco) The Rice One Simply Salt (crackers)
18. Great Value Gluten Free Wavy Original Potato chip
19. Great Value Peanut Butter
20. Great Value Picante Sauce
21. Herdez tortilla chips, white corn
22. Hummus is generally gluten and dairy free but when purchasing various flavors of hummus I would suggest checking the ingredient list as I found a few that stated milk.
23. Jif Peanut Butter
24. Skippy peanut butter
25. Joyva Tahini Creamy Puree Sesame Seeds
26. Kettle brand potato chips
27. Kind almond & coconut fruit and nut bar
28. KIND Gluten Free, Dairy free, yeast free Granola Bar
29. Kroger Creamy Peanut Butter
30. Kroger Natural Peanut Butter
31. Larabar Gluten Free Granola Bars
32. Lay's Potato Chips, Classic
33. Lets do gluten free ice cream cones

A COMPREHENSIVE GLUTEN & DAIRY FREE GROCERY LIST

34. Libre Naturals Granola Bars
35. Lucy's chocolate chip cookies
36. Lundberg Rice Cakes
37. MadeGood Crispy Squares
38. Manischewitz gluten free crackers, salted
39. maraNatha Creamy Coconut Almond Butter
40. Marshmallows, such as the ingredients in Jet~Puffed Marshmallows
41. Mozaics organic popped veggie & potato chips, BBQ
42. Mozaics organic popped veggie & potato chips, sea salt
43. Mission tortilla chips
44. Nuts and Seeds (all without seasonings)
45. On the border mixican grill café style tortilla chips
46. Paleo Thin USDA Organic Crackers
47. Peanut butter: most peanut butter is okay but check the label
48. PB2 Powdered Peanut Butter
49. Pik-Nik original shoestring potatoes
50. Plantain chips
51. Popcorn (no butter or cheese varieties)
52. Potato chips: potatoes are free of gluten and dairy. Just be careful of any added ingredients. Many have whey (a dairy) and/or barley malt flour, (a gluten), among other ingredients you will want to avoid. Some gluten and dairy free brands and varieties are in this list.
53. Pork Rinds: check the label if choosing a variety with seasoning
54. Pringles Sour cream & onion contains gluten and dairy!
55. Pringles Wavy Classic Salted
56. Pumpkin Seeds
57. Quaker Caramel or Apple Cinnamon Rice Cakes
58. Quaker Lightly Salted Rice Cakes
59. Rhythm superfoods naked beets chips
60. Roland Organic Tahini
61. Ruffles original potato chips
62. Sabra Classic Hummus
63. Sabra Roasted Pine Nut Hummus
64. Sabra Roasted Red Pepper Hummus

A COMPREHENSIVE GLUTEN & DAIRY FREE GROCERY LIST

65. Saffron road baked lentil chips
66. Sesmark Gluten Free Rice Thins, Brown Rice Crackers
67. Simple Mills Almond Flour Crackers
68. Simple truth organic blue corn tortilla chips
69. Simply7 Gluten Free Quinoa Curls
70. Simply7 Hummus Chips
71. Simply7 Kale Chips
72. SkinnyPop Popped Popcorn
73. Smuckers goober grape peanut butter & grape jelly stripes
74. Snyder's of Hanover Gluten Free Pretzels
75. So Natural Freeze Dried Strawberries
76. Sweet Lorens Cookie Dough Place & Bake Gluten Free Chocolate Chunk cookies
77. *"The better chip"* brand whole grain chips
78. Trader joe's barbeque popped ridges
79. Utz Potato Stix Shoestrings
80. Utz Pork Rinds, Plain (per the co., these are made in a plant that also mfg wheat)
81. Utz Potato Chips, Crab
82. Vans fire roasted veggie gluten free crackers
83. Welches Fruit Snacks
84. Wild Garden Hummus Dip, traditional, jalepeno, roasted garlic & sundried tomato variety.
85. Yummy earth gluten free strawberry licorice

A COMPREHENSIVE GLUTEN & DAIRY FREE GROCERY LIST

COOKIES AND SNACK CAKES

1. Annie's Gluten Free Chewy Granola Bars
2. Annie's Gluten Free Bunny Grahams
3. Emmy's Organics Gluten Free Vegan Cookies
4. Enjoy Life Gluten Free, Allergy Friendly Soft Baked Cookies
5. Enjoy Life Chocolate Bars: Soy free, nut free, gluten free, dairy free
6. Enjoy Life Crunchy Mini Cookies
7. Enjoy Life Gingerbread Spice Cookies
8. GluteNull Cookies (Lemon coconut, Hemp, Ginger Squares
9. Glutino Gluten Free Chocolate Chip Cookies (and other flavors!)
10. Glutino Wafers
11. Katz Heavenly Crème Cakes
12. Katz Mini Pies
13. Katz Raspberry tart
14. Katz Vanilla Cookies
15. KIND gluten free granola/snack bars (check the labels)
16. Kinnikinnick Gluten Free Animal Graham Cookies
17. Natures Bakery Fig Bars
18. Newman's Own Wheat Free Dairy Free Fig Newmans
19. Schar gluten free shortbread cookies
20. Schar Honeygrams Graham Style Crackers
21. Sweet Loren's Gluten Free (Dairy Free) Chocolate Chunk Place & Bake Cookie Dough
22. Tom & Luke Healthy Snack Balls
23. Trader joe's dark chocolate sunflower seed butter cups
24. Trader joe's mini peppermint meringues

SOUPS, BROTHS, SAUCE AND GRAVY

BROTH

1. Bouillon: most bouillon are gluten free, check the label
2. Broth: not all canned and boxed broth is gluten and dairy free! But broth, all broth, in and of itself, is gluten and dairy free.
3. Kettle & fire beef bone broth
4. Knorr Granulated Bouillon
5. Maggi Granulated Bouillon
6. Mayacamas Demi Glace Gluten Free Sauce Mix
7. More Than Gourmet Classic Roasted Vegetable Demi-Glace, Gluten Free
8. More Than Gourmet Glace De Canard Gold Roasted Duck Stock, Gluten Free
9. More Than Gourmet Glace De Veau Gold, Gluten Free Reduced Veal Stock
10. More Than Gourmet Glace De Volaille Gold Roasted Gluten Free Turkey Stock
11. More Than Gourmet Jus De Poulet Lie Gold Gluten Free
12. Roasted Chicken Demi-glace
13. Pacific organic Beef Broth
14. Pacific Organic Bone Broth, Chicken (box)
15. Pacific chicken broth
16. Pacific organic Mushroom Broth
17. Swanson Natural Goodness Broth: all varieties
18. Savory Choice Chicken Broth Concentrate
19. Savory Choice Liquid Beef Broth Concentrate
20. Simple truth organic broth

SOUP, CHILI, AND STEW

1. Amy's french country vegetable canned soup
2. Amy's organic soup chunky vegetable, canned
3. Amy's Organic Soups, Lentil (canned)
4. Amy's Thai Curry Sweet Potato Lentil canned soup
5. Dinty Moore Beef Stew
6. Dr. McDougalls Vegan Pad Thai Noodle Soup
7. **Gluten free Café' Chicken Noodle Soup**
8. Hormel Chili with Beans
9. Nona Lim Carrot Ginger Soup
10. Pacific organic Carrot Ginger Soup (box)
11. Pacific organic Creamy Butternut Squash Soup
12. Pacific organic Thai Sweet Potato Soup
13. Pacific organic Vegetable Lentil & Roasted Red Pepper soup (box)
14. Progresso Chicken & Wild Rice Soup's ingredients are gf/df. If you have issues with this product it may be due to possible cross-contamination.
15. Stagg Chili: not the Stagg Chili Country Brand, Turkey Ranchero or Laredo as they list wheat flour in the ingredients lists. Most Stagg Chili varieties are gluten and dairy free but a few will have the wheat flour in the ingredients lists. I have listed the varieties that do not have gluten.
16. Stagg: Classic Chili with or without beans
17. Stagg vegetable garden
18. Stagg chunkero
19. Stagg chili ranch house chicken chili with beans
20. Trader joe's organic hearty minestrone soup
21. Trader joe's organic pea soup
22. Wolf Brand Chili with beans

GRAVY

1. OrgraN Gluten Free Gravy Mix
2. Pacific Organic Vegan Mushroom Gravy (box)
3. Road's End Organics delicious golden quick gravy packet

SAUCE

1. Chi-chi's enchilada sauce
2. Classico pasta sauce (except cheese varieties)
3. Dei Fratelli All Purpose Italian Sauce
4. Dei fratelli pizza sauce
5. Eden Organic Spaghetti Sauce heirloom variety
6. Emeril's roasted gaaahlic pasta sauce
7. Francesco Rinaldi Original Recipe Spaghetti Sauce
8. Great value traditional pasta sauce (not the cheese varieties
9. Hatch gluten free green chili enchilada sauce
10. Hatch gluten free red enchilada sauce
11. Hunts Traditional Pasta Sauce
12. Las palmas green chile enchilada sauce
13. Mezzetta Napa Valley Homemade Marinara sauce
14. New primal marinade and cooking sauce, citrus herb
15. Nonna pia's balsamic glaze – strawberry fig
16. Organic Amy's Pasta Sauce
17. Organico bello organic marinara organic pasta sauce
18. Prego traditional pasta Sauce
19. Rao's homemade marinara sauce
20. Ying's sweet & sour sauce
21. Yo Mama's Marinara

SPICES & SEASONINGS

> *Most extracts are gluten free. Take a quick glance at the ingredients list.*

1. Ac'cent flavor enhancer
2. Adams Imitation Butter Flavoring Extract (not all butter extract or flavoring is gluten and dairy free so please check the label)
3. All Single spices, but not blends
4. Allspice
5. Almond Extract
6. Alum
7. Anise Extract
8. Apple Pie Spice
9. Banana extract
10. Bay leaves
11. Black pepper
12. Bragg Liquid Aminos All Purpose Seasoning
13. Butter Buds Sprinkles All Natural Butter Flavor granules: per the company web site this is dairy free.
14. Cayenne
15. Chi-chi's fiesta restaurante seasoning mix packet
16. Chili powder
17. Cilantro
18. Cinnamon
19. Cloves
20. Coconut extract
21. Cream of Tartar
22. Cumin
23. Dill
24. Emeri's original essence
25. Enjoy Life Lentil Chips
26. Food coloring
27. Garam masala
28. Garlic powder
29. Garlic salt

A COMPREHENSIVE GLUTEN & DAIRY FREE GROCERY LIST

30. Gourmet garden stir-in paste ginger (the Gourmet Garden stir in paste gluten free garlic has milk listed as an ingredient)
31. Granulated garlic
32. Great Value Real Bacon Pieces
33. Grill mates applewood rub
34. Ground ginger
35. Himalayan pink salt
36. Lawry's seasoned salt
37. Lemon extracts
38. Lemon pepper
39. Liquid smoke
40. Louisiana fish fry crawfish, crab and shrimp boil, 5oz bags
41. Mace
42. Maple extract
43. McCormick Bag 'n Season pork chops cooking & seasoning mix
44. McCormick Cake Batter Flavor
45. Mccormick fajitas seasoning mix
46. McCormick gluten free taco seasoning mix
47. mcCormick sloppy joes seasoning mix
48. Mint
49. Mint Extract
50. Montreal Chicken seasoning
51. Montreal steak seasoning (McCormick Grill Mates)
52. Mrs. Dash Original Blend salt-free
53. Mrs. Wages all natural guacamole seasoning mix packet (many guacamole mix seasoning packets are gluten free but have milk in the ingredients list. Mrs. Wages is a gluten and dairy free mix. Check other brands to be sure it is gluten and dairy free both, before purchasing.
54. Nomu Egyptian Dukkah
55. Nutmeg
56. Old Bay Seasoning
57. Onion powder
58. Orange extract
59. Orange Peel
60. Oregano
61. Paprika (a nightshade)
62. Parsley
63. Pepper
64. Poppy Seed
65. Red Pepper (a nightshade)

A COMPREHENSIVE GLUTEN & DAIRY FREE GROCERY LIST

66. Rum extract
67. Salt
68. Sea salt
69. Strawberry extract
70. Stubbs chili fixins cookin sauce mix
71. Thai kitchen gluten free green curry paste
72. Thyme
73. Tones lemon pepper seasoning blend
74. Tones italian seasoning blend
75. Tones roasted garlic & herb seasonning
76. Tones rosemary garlic seasoning blend
77. Tony chachere's creole seasoning
78. turmeric
79. Vanilla extract
80. Watkins Imitation Butter Extract
81. Watkins red velvet flavor
82. Weber bold chipotle seasoning
83. Weber gourmet burger seasoning
84. Weber honey garlic rub
85. Weber kick'n chicken seasoning
86. Whole Vanilla Bean
87. Zatarain's new orleans style blackened seasoning

SWEETENERS

1. Agave nectar
2. Beet sugar
3. Brown Sugar
4. Cane sugar
5. Coconut Sugar
6. Equal
7. Honey
8. Lundberg sweet dreams brown rice syrup
9. Molasses
10. Pure Cane Sugar
11. Splenda
12. Starbucks caramel syrup
13. Starbucks Hazelnut syrup
14. Stevia
15. Sugar-in-the Raw
16. Torani Flavoring Syrups
17. White sugar
18. Xylitol

A COMPREHENSIVE GLUTEN & DAIRY FREE GROCERY LIST

VEGETABLES: PRODUCE

1. Acorn squash
2. Artichokes
3. Arugula
4. Avocado
5. Basil
6. Bean sprouts
7. Beats
8. Bell peppers
9. Bok choy
10. Broccoli
11. Brussels sprouts
12. Cabbage
13. Carrots
14. Cauliflower
15. Celery
16. Celery root
17. Chayote
18. Chives
19. Cilantro
20. Collard greens
21. Corn
22. Cucumber
23. Dill
24. Edamame
25. Eggplant
26. Endive
27. Fennel
28. Fiddlehead
29. Garlic
30. Ginger root
31. Grape leaves
32. Green beans
33. Green Giant Riced Veggies, Cauliflower & Sweet Potato (frozen)
34. Green giant riced veggies cauliflower medley (frozen)
35. Green giant veggie spirals zucchini (frozen)
36. Horseradish root
37. Jicama
38. Kale

A COMPREHENSIVE GLUTEN & DAIRY FREE GROCERY LIST

39. Kohlrabi
40. Leeks
41. Lemongrass
42. Lotus root
43. Mushrooms
44. Mustard greens
45. Okra
46. Onions
47. Oregano
48. Parsley
49. Parsnips
50. Peppers
51. plantains
52. Potatoes: all
53. Pumpkin
54. Radicchio
55. Radishes
56. Rosemary
57. Rutabaga
58. Sage
59. Sea vegetables
60. Seaweed
61. Snow peas
62. Spaghetti squash
63. Spinach
64. Sugar snap peas
65. Swiss chard
66. tarragon
67. Tofu
68. Tomatillo
69. tomato
70. Turnip greens
71. Turnips
72. Yellow squash
73. Yuca
74. Zucchini

TIPS FOR HEALTHY GROCERY SHOPPING

Produce: When buying produce don't get over zealous. Be sure to have meals planned to use the produce and then only buy just enough produce to last you the next 7 days.

Moisture is what will cause your produce to go bad before you get the chance to eat it. I find most produce can last up to two full weeks by keeping it dry and in an airtight container or ziploc baggie. Don't wash your produce until you are going to prepare and serve it. And then, only wash the amount you will be preparing and serving.

The most common advice I give out is if you buy it, plan on eating in the first 5 days or yes, it may very well go bad.

There are some items in the produce department you can bring home and simply place in a jar, container or freezer bag and freeze for months. Here are some of those foods:

1. Garlic bulbs
2. Ginger root
3. Horseradish root
4. Red or purple grapes (not green): wash and remove the stems before freezing.
5. The juice from citrus
6. Bananas! Slice really, really thin (this is very important). Freeze, and then you can put that in your food chopper or food processor and make what some call a "n'ice cream". It does take some patience to get it going in the food processor at first, but hang in there and you will have the consistency of actual ice cream. Eat it as is or add cocoa and sugar, strawberries, or vanilla and a can of chilled coconut milk.
7. Berries! Wash and allow to dry before freezing.
8. Tomatoes. Just dice them up or puree them. No need to cook them. After freezing you can use them just like you would canned tomatoes.
9. Celery. If you find your celery got a little limp instead of throwing it away dice it up and freeze. No cooking necessary. Great to add to soups, sauces, and smoothies.

10. Cranberries. Every year when the fresh bag of cranberries come out I buy several bags and put them in the freezer. First place them in a freezer bag or container.
11. Carrots. If your carrots have become soft but have not started turned black slice them up, boil them until soft. Drain. Place the carrots in your blender or food processor to puree. Add just enough fresh water to get it going. You want the consistency of gravy. Freeze flat in freezer bags and then stack or use freezer safe containers or canning jars. Pureed carrots is very healthy. I eat heated pureed carrots two or three times a week for breakfast in the winter. I heat and add a little honey, cinnamon and dairy free butter. I also make no'mato sauce with mine which depending on the type of vinegar and spices I add is used for making lasagna, chili, tacos, pizza sauce, tomato soup and sloppy joes without using nightshades.
12. Green Beans: snip the ends, wash and par-boil. Once cooled completely place in a freezer safe container or baggie. For best results on taste, boil in salted water.

RESOURCES FOR MORE INFORMATION

www.celiac.com: This site has gobs of information you will find helpful even if you are not celiac. Great support and information for those avoiding gluten.

Check out my web site for even more shopping lists, recipes and more:
www.glutenfree-dairyfree-recipes.com

www.bobsredmill.com/shop/gluten-free.html

www.katzglutenfree.com/

www.cup4cup.com/

www.namastefoods.com/

www.kingarthurflour.com

www.pamelasproducts.com/

www.schaer.com

www.kinnikinnick.com

www.simplemills.com

www.ancientharvest.com/

www.followyourheart.com

www.amys.com

www.rightfoods.com

www.pacificfoods.com

www.udisglutenfree.com

www.daiyafoods.com/

Paula has written a few gluten and dairy free cookbooks:

Gluten and Dairy Free Living Recipes
Ebook and paperback

52 Low Carb Gluten and Dairy Free Chicken Recipes
Ebook and paperback

Summer Body Recipes: gluten and dairy free recipes with a focus on low carb ingredients.

Find all of her books on her web site
www.glutenfree-dairyfree-recipes.com
or my Amazon author's page:
www.amazon.com/author/paula-c-henderson

A COMPREHENSIVE GLUTEN & DAIRY FREE GROCERY LIST

Printed in Great Britain
by Amazon